CALISTHENICS ESSENTIALS

A Beginner's Guide to Mastering Bodyweight, Strengthen, and Energize Your Body Without the Need for Gym Equipment With 30-days Calisthenic challenge and 7-days meal plan

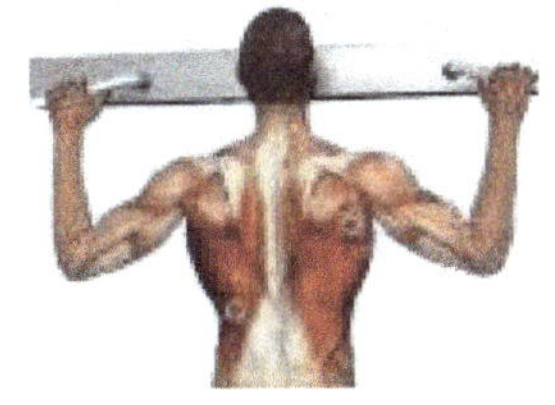

RICHARD E. MARSHALL

CONTENTS:

INTRODUCTION

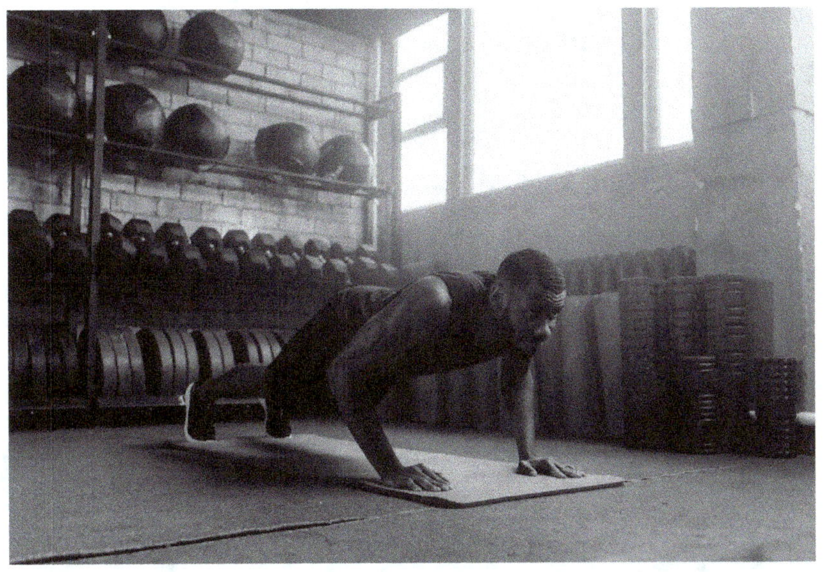

Brief Overview of Calisthenics

The muscular man at your gym who can lift his entire upper body above a pull-up bar is performing a muscle-up and calisthenics. The person you watched on YouTube who made himself into a human flag by holding his body parallel to the ground is also performing calisthenics, as is the guy you saw doing dips in the park.

The phrase calisthenics is derived from the Greek terms 'Kalos' (beauty) and 'Stenos' (strength).

Originally intended to promote health, 'and thereby securing beauty and strength' in schoolchildren, calisthenics has grown into a training style with many similarities to gymnastics. However, unlike gymnastics, it may be done outside and is referred to as a "street workout."

Most individuals learn about calisthenics by watching someone do an advanced version of it. The guy they saw was presumably Hannibal Lanham, also known as Hannibal for King, whose form of calisthenics, which he practiced in parks throughout Queens, New York, brought the discipline to the attention of millions.

The Benefits of Calisthenics

Calisthenics, which has its roots in ancient Greek training methods, has evolved into a modern fitness discipline that focuses on mastering motions and regulating one's body through space.

Calisthenics, in essence, is a diversified set of exercises that require little to no equipment, making it an accessible and adaptable type of training. Calisthenics offers a progressive progression ideal for persons of varying fitness levels, ranging from fundamental motions like squats and push-ups to advanced abilities like muscle-ups and handstands.

Minimal Equipment Required

One of the most significant benefits of calisthenics is that they can be performed anywhere, without the need for pricey equipment or gym subscriptions. To get a fantastic exercise, all you need is your body and some free space.

Enhances Functional Strength

Calisthenics motions are imitations of natural bodily movements such as pushing, pulling, squatting, and leaping. This sort of exercise promotes functional strength, which aids in daily tasks and athletic performance.

Boosts flexibility and mobility

Calisthenics demand a broad range of motion, which improves flexibility and mobility. This form of exercise can help lower the chance of injury and enhance general health over time.

Increases lean muscle mass

Calisthenics exercises work many muscle groups at the same time, resulting in a more toned and defined body.

Consistent exercise can help you gain lean muscle mass and enhance your body composition.

Offers a Full-Body Workout

Calisthenics workouts frequently include complex motions that engage numerous muscle groups at the same time. As a result, you may receive a full-body workout in a short period of time, making it an efficient and effective type of exercise.

Scalability for People of All Fitness Levels

Calisthenics, whether you're a novice or an established fitness lover, provides for progressive improvement. Exercise modifications and adaptations make it suitable for people of varying fitness levels.

Improved Mental Focus

Mastering calisthenics techniques demands concentration, focus, and a mind-body connection. This mental involvement can boost cognitive performance and reduce stress.

Calisthenics Versus Weights

Still not ready to abandon your weighted workouts? That's OK, but have you ever considered transitioning from calisthenics to those kinds of workouts? Calisthenics may serve as a foundation for any other strength-building exercise, including bodybuilding and CrossFit.

'To me, everyone out there in the gym trying to bench press, trying to do curls, if you can't pull your body up in a pull-up, if you can't push your body up in a press-up, you have no right to be lifting weights. That is not to argue that utilizing weights and bulking up is not permitted in calisthenics. Weights can be employed as long as your body moves in natural patterns.

Studies About Calisthenics

It has been found that training in calisthenics has actual advantages. The 2017 study, 'The effects of a calisthenics training intervention on posture, strength, and body composition,' conducted by scientists from the Sport and Exercise Sciences research unit at the University of Palermo, Italy, discovered that calisthenics training is a "effective training solution to improve posture, strength, and body composition without the use of any major training equipment."

The males in the research were separated into two groups of 28. For eight weeks, one group did calisthenics while the other remained with their regular fitness routines. After eight weeks, all participants were subjected to a body composition analysis, a posture evaluation, a handgrip test, and press-up and pull-up tests.

The males who trained in calisthenics improved their posture and reduced their fat mass, while their ability to perform press-ups and pull-ups rose, despite the fact that their calisthenics training did not contain these specific activities. The group who proceeded with their usual training habits, on the other hand, did not much improve on what they could achieve before the eight weeks began.

CHAPTER 1

Getting Started

Examining Your Fitness Level

Before diving into the realm of calisthenics, it's critical to analyze your present fitness level honestly. This assessment acts as a baseline, allowing you to personalize your training regimen to your unique requirements and skills.

Self-Assessment

Begin by thinking about your daily routine, lifestyle, and previous workout experiences. Consider any injuries or health issues that may have an impact on your training. Examine your strengths and shortcomings, noting any areas that require further attention.

Physical Examination

If feasible, schedule a physical exam with a healthcare practitioner or fitness specialist. By recognizing any limits or pre-existing problems that may affect your calisthenics journey, this stage can provide you important insights into your general health.

Baseline Fitness Tests

Assess your endurance, flexibility, and strength with baseline fitness tests. Push-ups, squats, planks, and timed runs are common tests. Recording your initial performance helps you to measure your improvement and celebrate your accomplishments as you grow.

Setting Realistic Goals

Once you've determined your starting place, the next critical step is to create reasonable and attainable goals. Throughout your calisthenics journey, goals give direction, motivation, and a feeling of purpose.

Short-Term Goals

Start with short-term goals that can be accomplished in a few weeks to a few months. If you can now perform five push-ups, a short-term objective may be to go to 10. These small victories keep you motivated and focused.

Long-Term goals

Long-term objectives, which often cover several months to a year, give a larger perspective. Think of where you want to go in terms of fitness at the conclusion of this period. Long-term objectives influence your general trajectory, whether it's learning a difficult calisthenics technique, obtaining a certain body composition, or finishing a comprehensive exercise regimen.

SMART goals

When creating objectives, use the SMART criteria: Specific, Measurable, Achievable, Relevant, and Time-bound. A SMART goal may be something like, "Increase the duration of my plank from 30 seconds to 2 minutes within the next 8 weeks."

Developing a Reliable Routine

Consistency is the foundation of calisthenics growth. Creating a regimen that fits your objectives and lifestyle is essential for long-term success. When creating your training routine, keep the following factors in mind:

Frequency

Figure out how many days a week you can dedicate to doing calisthenics. For novices, consistency is more crucial than intensity. A fair method is to begin with 2-3 days per week and progressively increase.

Progressive Overload

Use the progressive overload theory to gradually increase the intensity of your workouts. As your strength develops, you can increase the number of repetitions, sets, or incorporate more difficult variants of exercises.

Workout Balance

Create a well-rounded plan that targets various muscle groups. To achieve balanced growth, use pushing, pulling, and leg movements. In order to improve general athleticism, include both strength-focused activities and skill practice.

Rest and Recovery

Acknowledge the value of rest days in your schedule. Your muscles require time to heal and adapt to the strain of exercise. Overtraining can cause tiredness, increase the likelihood of injury, and impede growth.

Warm-up and cool-down are essential.

Warming up and cooling down are sometimes overlooked aspects of an exercise regimen. They do, however, play an important role in injury prevention, performance enhancement, and overall exercise enjoyment.

Warm-up

A good warm-up gets your body ready for the physical demands of exercise. It enhances joint flexibility by increasing blood flow to the muscles, raising core body temperature, and increasing blood flow to the muscles. A dynamic warm-up that includes movements like jumping jacks, bodyweight squats, and arm circles prepares your body for the activity ahead.

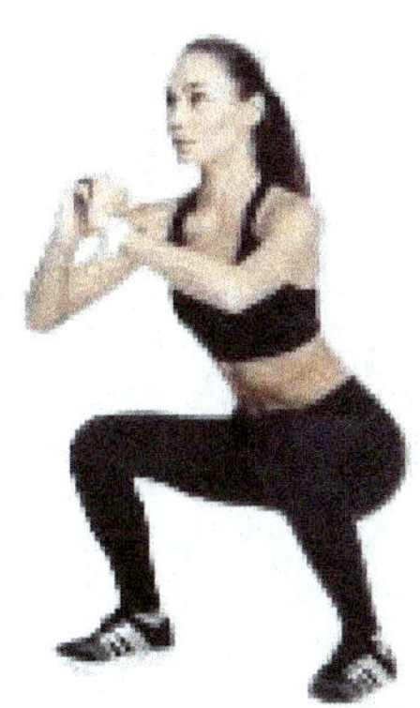

Cool Down

The cool-down phase is equally vital for shifting your body from a state of intensive activity to one of rest. It facilitates a steady reduction in heart rate and helps to minimize muscular soreness. Incorporate static stretches into your cool-down practice, concentrating on the muscle areas you focused on throughout the exercise.

Mind-Body Connection

Both the warm-up and cool-down phases allow for the development of a mind-body connection. Use this time to mentally prepare for your workout or to reflect on your success. Similarly, during the cool-down, express thanks for the time and work you've put into your health.

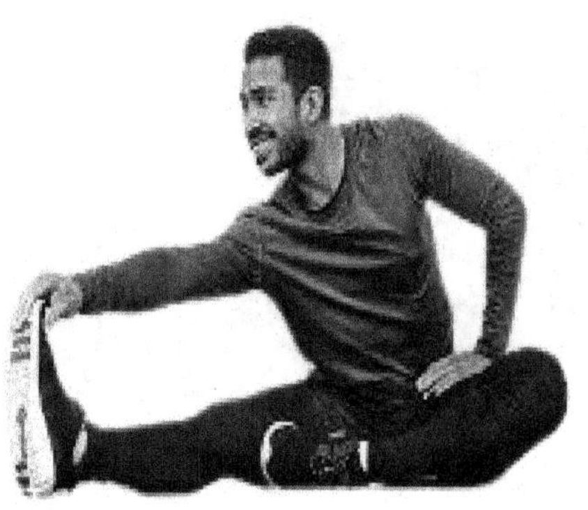

CHAPTER 2

Foundation Exercises

Bodyweight Squats:

- Place your feet shoulder-width apart.
- Bend your knees and drop your hips to squat.
- Keep your back straight and your chest up.
- 3 sets of 10-15 repetitions

Push-Ups:

- Start in the plank posture.
- Bend your elbows to lower your body.
- Push yourself back up.
- 3 sets of 5-10 repetitions

Pull-Ups:

- Hang from a bar with your hands facing out.
- Raise your body till your chin is above the bar.
- Lower yourself back down.
- Reps: 3 sets of 3-5 reps (assisted if necessary).

Inverted Rows:

- Lie down under a bar and grasp it with an overhand hold.
- Draw your chest up to the bar.
- 3 sets of 8-12 repetitions

Lunges:

- Take a step forward with one leg.
- Bend both knees and lower your hips.
- Alternate the legs.
- 3 sets of ten sets of reps per leg

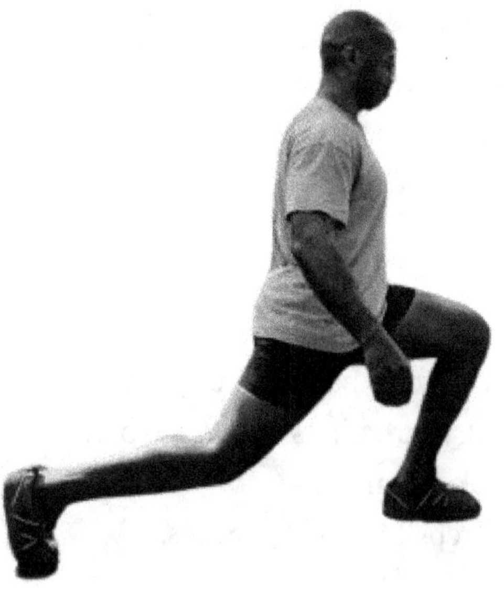

Dips:

- Make use of parallel bars.
- Bend your elbows to lower your body.
- Push yourself back up.
- 3 sets of 5-10 repetitions

Plank:

- Maintain a push-up position with a straight line from your head to your heels.
- 3 sets of 30-60 seconds each

Mountain Climbers:

- Bring one knee to your chest from a plank posture.
- Rapidly switch legs.
- 3 sets of 20 repetitions (10 reps per leg)

Superman Exercise:

- Lift your arms and legs off the ground while lying face down.
- Stretch your glutes.

- 3 sets of 12-15 repetitions

Calf Raises:

- Place your feet on a level surface.
- Raise your heels to your toes and then drop them back down.
- 3 sets of 15-20 repetitions

Tricep Dips:

- Sit on the edge of a bench.
- Put your hands beside your hips.
- Push yourself back up after lowering your body.
- 3 sets of 8-12 repetitions

Bodyweight Rows:

- Position yourself at an angle using a solid bar.
- Pull your chest up to the bar.
- 3 sets of 8-12 repetitions

Side Plank:

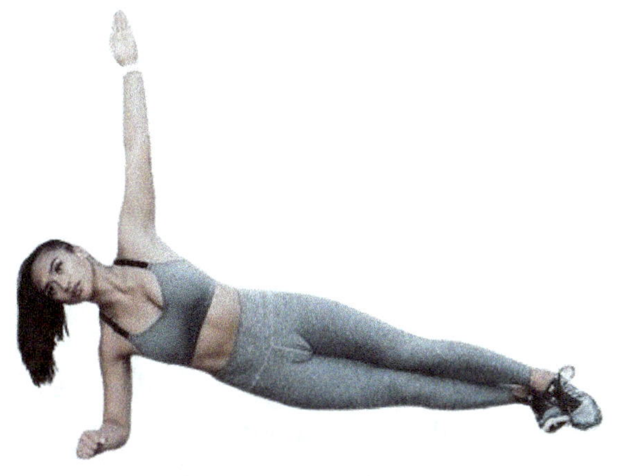

- Lie on your side, elevate your torso, and balance on your forearm.
- Make a straight line from your head to your heels.
- 3 sets of 20-30 seconds on each side

Jumping Jacks:

- Begin with your feet together.
- Jump with your legs open and your arms up high.
- 3 sets of 30 seconds reps

Hollow Body Hold:

- Lift your legs and upper body off the ground while lying on your back.
- Keep a hollow posture.
- 3 sets of 20-30 seconds each

Box Jumps:

- Place yourself in front of a strong box.
- Take a step up and then back down on it.
- 3 sets of 10-15 repetitions

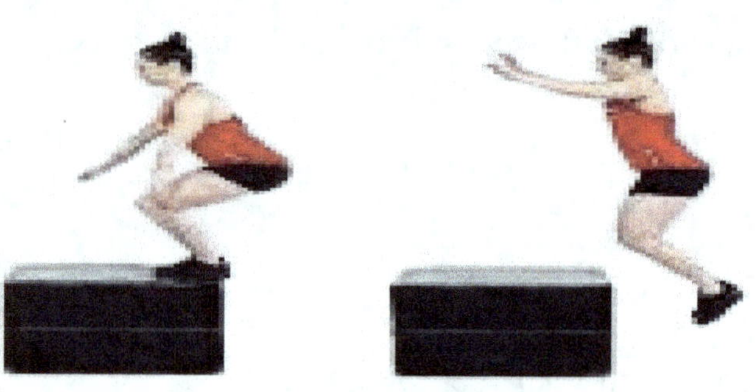

Russian Twists:

- Sit on the ground and lean gently back.
- Twist your torso on either side while contacting the ground.
- 3 sets of 15-20 repetitions on each side

Flutter Kicks:

- Lie down on your back and raise your legs off the ground.
- Perform quick, tiny kicks.
- 3 sets of 30 seconds reps

Seated Leg Raises:

- Sit on the edge of a bench and lean slightly back.
- Raise your legs to your chest.
- 3 sets of 12-15 repetitions

Burpees:

- Squat down from a standing posture.

- Perform a push-up after kicking your feet back into a plank position.
- Return your feet to the ground and then spring up.
- 3 sets of 8-12 repetitions

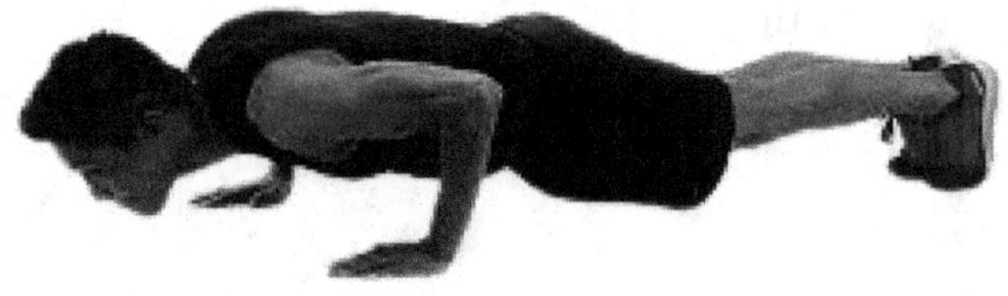

CHAPTER 3

Building Strength

Pike Push-Ups:

- **Target:** Shoulders, triceps, upper chest
- Begin in a downward dog position, drop your head to the ground, and push back up.
- 3 sets of 8-12 repetitions

Diamond Push-Ups:

- **Target:** Triceps, inner chest
- **Steps:** Form a diamond formation beneath your chest with your hands, lower your body, and push back up.
- 3 sets of 8-12 repetitions

Wide Grip Pull-Ups:

- **Target:** Lats, biceps, upper back
- **Steps:** Perform pull-ups with a grip that is broader than shoulder width.

- 3 sets of 5-8 repetitions

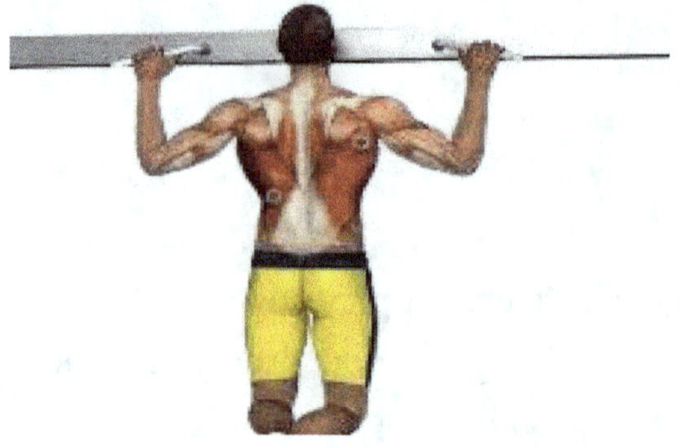

Commando Pull-Ups:

- **Target:** Lats, biceps, shoulders
- **Steps:** Pull yourself up towards one hand, then switch to the opposite side and repeat.
- 3 sets of 5-8 reps on each side

Box Pistol Squats:

- **Target:** Quadriceps, hamstrings, glutes
- **Steps:** Stand on one leg in front of a box, squat, and then stand back up.
- 3 sets of 8-10 repetitions per leg.

L-Sit Progression:

- **Target:** Core, hip flexors
- **Steps:** Sit on the floor, elevate your legs, and tuck them in before straightening them.
- 3 sets of 10-20 seconds each

Tuck Jumps:

- **Target:** Legs (quadriceps, hamstrings, glutes)
- **Steps:** Jump quickly while pulling your knees up to your chest.
- 3 sets of 15-20 repetitions

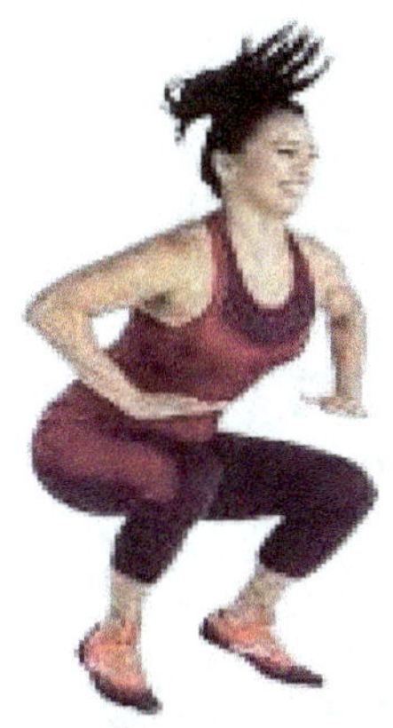

Decline Push-Ups:

- **Target:** Upper chest, shoulders
- **Steps:** Place your feet on a raised place and do push-ups with your hands on the ground.
- 3 sets of 8-12 repetitions

Negative Pull-Ups:

- **Target:** Building pulling strength
- **Steps:** Jump up to the bar and slowly drop yourself down.
- 3 sets of 3-5 repetitions

Step-Ups:

- **Target:** Legs (quadriceps, hamstrings, glutes)
- Steps: With one leg, step up onto a bench or strong surface and step back down.
- 3 sets of ten repetitions per leg

Assisted One-Arm Push-Ups:

- **Target:** Chest, triceps, shoulders

- **Steps:** Place one hand on an elevated platform and do push-ups with help.
- 3 sets of 5-8 reps on each side

Chin-Ups:

- **Target:** Biceps, lats, upper back
- **Steps:** Pull-ups should be done with a supinated (palms facing you) grip.
- 3 sets of 5-8 repetitions

Core Strengthening

Hanging Leg Raises:

- **Target:** Lower abs, hip flexors
- **Steps:** Hang from a bar and raise your legs to the ceiling.
- 3 sets of 10-15 repetitions

Plank Variations:

- **Target:** Core
- **Steps:** Include variants of high plank, low plank, and side plank.
- 3 sets of 30-60 seconds for each variation.

Windshield Wipers:

- **Target:** Obliques
- **Steps:** Lie on your back and elevate your legs, rotating them side to side.
- 3 sets of 12-15 repetitions on each side

Dragon Flags:

- **Target:** Abdominals, lower back
- **Steps:** Lie on your back, raise your legs and hips, and then lower them without contacting the ground.
- 3 sets of 8-12 repetitions

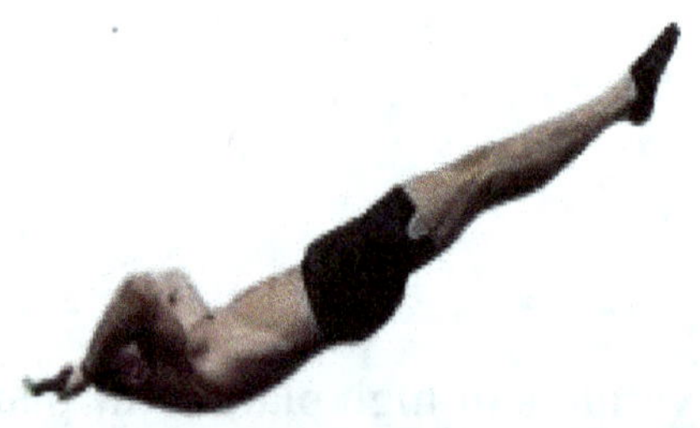

Russian Twists with Medicine Ball:

- **Target:** Obliques, abdominals
- **Steps:** Sit on the ground, grasp a medicine ball, and twist your torso on each side while touching the ground.
- 3 sets of 15-20 repetitions on each side

Bicycle Crunches:

- **Target:** Obliques, abdominals
- **Steps:** Lie on your back and pedal by bringing your knee to the opposite elbow.
- 3 sets of 20-30 repetitions (10-15 reps per leg)

Leg Raises:

- **Target:** Lower abs
- **Steps:** Lie on your back, raise your legs to the ceiling, and then lower them without hitting the ground.
- 3 sets of 12-15 repetitions

Hollow Body Rocks:

- **Target:** Abdominals, lower back
- **Steps:** Lie on your back and rock back and forth while lifting your legs and upper torso.
- 3 sets of 15-20 repetitions

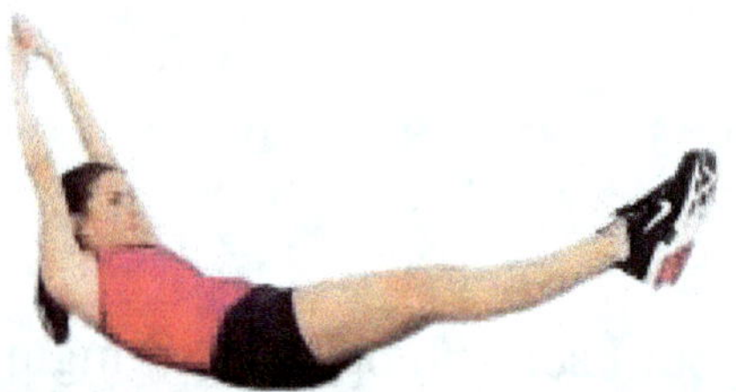

CHAPTER 4

Full Body Workouts routine

Warm-Up:

Jumping Jacks:

Perform a 2-minute warm-up to raise your heart rate and warm up your entire body.

Dynamic Lunges:

Step forward and alternate legs into a lunge stance. Do two sets of ten lunges per leg.

Arm Circles:

For 1 minute, rotate your arms forward and backward in a circular manner.

Main Workout:

Bodyweight Squats:

- **Target:** Lower body (quads, hamstrings, glutes)

- **Steps:** Stand with your feet shoulder-width apart, squat, then stand back up.
- 3 sets of 15 repetitions

Push-Ups:

- **Target:** Chest, shoulders, triceps
- **Steps:** Perform normal push-ups while maintaining perfect technique.
- 3 sets of 10 repetitions

Pull-Ups or Inverted Rows:

- **Target:** Upper back, biceps
- **Steps:** Select the option that best matches your current level of fitness.
- 3 sets of 5-8 repetitions

Dips:

- **Target:** Chest, triceps, shoulders
- **Steps:** Use parallel bars or strong furniture for the steps.
- 3 sets of 8-12 repetitions

Plank to Downward Dog:

- **Target:** Core, shoulders, hamstrings
- **Steps:** Begin in a plank position, then elevate your hips to form an inverted V and return to the plank position.
- 3 sets of 12 repetitions

Box Jumps:

- **Target:** Legs (quads, hamstrings, glutes)
- **Step 1:** Climb atop a solid box or platform.
- 3 sets of 10 repetitions

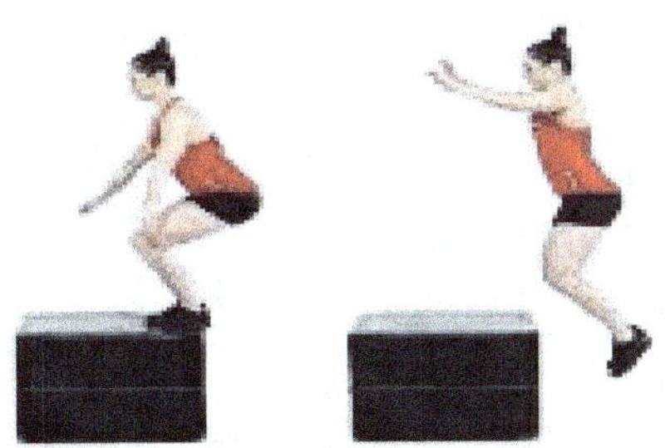

Russian Twists with a Twist:

- **Target:** Obliques, abdominals
- **Steps:** Sit on the ground, hold a weight or medicine ball in your hands, and rotate your body while elevating your feet off the ground.
- 3 sets of 15 repetitions on each side

Burpees:

- **Target:** Full body, cardiovascular system
- **Steps:** Squat, kick your feet back, execute a push-up, hop your feet back in, and jump up.
- 3 sets of 8-10 repetitions

L-Sit Progression:

- **Target:** Core, hip flexors
- **Steps:** Sit on the ground, elevate your legs, and tuck them in before straightening them.
- 3 sets of 15-20 seconds each

Cool down:

Child's Pose:

Stretch and relax your lower back and shoulders for 1 minute.

Downward Dog Stretch:

Stretch your hamstrings and calves by holding for 30 seconds.

Forward Bend While Seated:

While sitting, reach for your toes and hold for 30 seconds to stretch your hamstrings.

Cat-Cow Stretch:

To mobilize your spine, perform for 1 minute.

Side-Lying Thoracic Rotations:

Lie on one side and rotate your upper body for 30 seconds on each side.

Flexibility and Mobility:

Hip Flexor Stretch:

To stretch your hip flexors, hold for 30 seconds per leg.

Dynamic Leg Swings:

To develop hip flexibility, do two sets of 15 swings for each leg.

Wrist Mobility Workouts:

To enhance wrist flexibility, circle your wrists clockwise and counterclockwise for 1 minute.

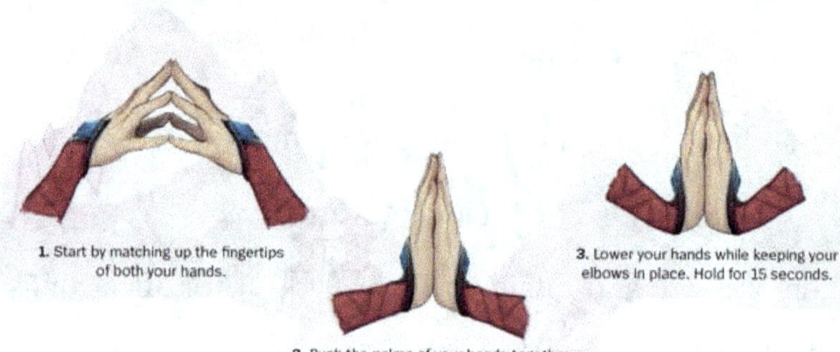

CHAPTER 5

The Symbiosis of Yoga and Calisthenics

1. Mind-Body Connection

Yoga Perspective: Yoga promotes the unity of mind, body, and spirit. Yoga practice includes mindful movement and breath awareness.

Calisthenics Integration: Yoga's mind-body connection complements calisthenics by improving precision, form, and purpose in each action.

2. Range of Motion and Flexibility

Yoga Perspective: Yoga postures promote muscle and joint elongation by cultivating flexibility.

Calisthenics Integration: Yoga's increased flexibility assists in performing calisthenics motions with a complete range of motion, lowering the risk of injury and improving overall performance.

3. Breathing Methods

Yoga Perspective: Pranayama, or breath control, is a fundamental part of yoga practice that promotes deep and aware breathing.

Calisthenics Integration: Including yogic breathing methods improves respiratory efficiency during calisthenics, optimizing oxygen transport to muscles and increasing endurance.

4. Core Stability and Strength

Yoga Perspective: Many yoga positions demand core engagement, which builds strength and stability.

Calisthenics Integration: Yoga builds a strong core, which helps with posture, balance, and strength in calisthenics movements like planks and leg lifts.

Practical Integration Techniques

1. Pre-Workout Yoga Flow

Begin your calisthenics workout with a vigorous yoga sequence that includes sun salutations and positions that target main muscle groups. This prepares the body for the physical demands of calisthenics.

2. Yoga Stretch After Workout

Finish your calisthenics workout with some yoga poses. Poses such as Downward Dog, Cobra, and Pigeon Stretch aid in the release of stress, the prevention of muscular stiffness, and the enhancement of flexibility.

3. Restorative Yoga on Days Off

Rest days should be reserved for restorative yoga sessions. Gentle postures and deep stretches help with recuperation, tired muscles, and overall well-being.

4. Movement Mindfulness

Using yoga concepts, incorporate awareness into your calisthenics exercise. Concentrate on the quality of each movement, keep your breath in check, and build a present-moment attitude.

Personal Experiences: The marriage of yoga and calisthenics has been physically and mentally transforming in my path. Yoga's increased flexibility has helped me to complete difficult calisthenics movements, and the awareness I've learned on the mat has transferred into better attention during exercises. The mutually beneficial interaction between the two activities has not only improved my physical ability but also given a safe haven for mental resilience and equilibrium.

When yoga and calisthenics are intelligently combined,
they produce a harmonic alliance that surpasses the
confines of standard workout regimens. The combination
of strength, flexibility, and mindfulness provides a holistic
approach to well-being, cultivating a body that moves with
grace, strength, and intention.

CHAPTER 6

Nutritional Guidelines

Peak performance in calisthenics is based not just on intense training, but also on a well-balanced and smart approach to diet. I highlight the importance of adequate nutrition in promoting strength, endurance, and general well-being as a certified fitness expert with vast experience in both calisthenics training and nutritional science.

Macronutrients and Micronutrients as the Foundation

1. Protein:

Professional Insight: Protein is essential for muscle repair and development. Protein intake of 1.6 to 2.2 grams per kilogram of body weight is critical for calisthenics aficionados.

Personal Experience: Including lean protein sources like chicken, fish, tofu, and lentils in every meal has really aided my muscle recuperation and strength growth.

2. Carbohydrates:

Professional Insight: Carbohydrates are the major energy source for calisthenics workouts. Complex carbs, such as those found in whole grains, fruits, and vegetables, provide long-lasting energy for intense workouts.

Personal Experience: Eating complex carbohydrates before exercises gives me the endurance I need to get through hard calisthenics programs.

3. Fats:

Professional Insight: Healthy fats, such as those found in avocados, almonds, and olive oil, are essential for hormone synthesis and joint health. The importance of balancing omega-3 and omega-6 fatty acids cannot be overstated.

Personal Experience: Incorporating a range of healthy fats has improved my joint flexibility and general well-being, both of which are necessary for negotiating difficult gymnastics motions.

4. Micronutrients:

Professional Insight: Vitamin D, calcium, and magnesium are essential vitamins and minerals that play important roles in bone health and muscular function. A well-balanced diet rich in colorful fruits and vegetables guarantees adequate micronutrient intake.

Personal Experience: Eating a variety of fruits and vegetables has not only improved my immune system but also allowed for faster recuperation between strenuous calisthenics workouts.

Hydration and Nutrient Timing

1. Pre-Exercise Nutrition:

Professional Insight: Consuming a healthy breakfast 2-3 hours before a calisthenics workout guarantees that you have the energy to last. Including a variety of carbohydrates, proteins, and fats promotes peak performance.

Personal Experience: A pre-workout breakfast of chicken and quinoa with mixed veggies has regularly powered my workouts without creating pain.

2. Hydration During Workout:

Professional Insight: It is critical to stay hydrated when performing calisthenics. Drinking water throughout the workout helps to avoid dehydration, muscular cramps, and weariness.

Personal Experience: I've seen a significant improvement in my endurance and attention by sipping water throughout calisthenics rests.

3. Post-Workout Nutrition:

Professional Insight: The post-workout time is crucial for restoring glycogen reserves and commencing muscle regeneration. It is best to have a combination of protein and carbs within 30-60 minutes.

Personal Experience: My go-to post-workout meal is a protein shake with a banana, which provides rapid and efficient nutritional replacement.

Considerations for Supplementation

1. Protein Supplements:

Professional Insight: Protein supplements, such as whey or plant-based protein powders, can be useful for achieving protein requirements, particularly for people with greater protein requirements.

Personal Experience: On hectic days, I mix a protein drink to ensure I fulfill my daily protein objectives.

2. Omega-3 Fatty Acids:

Professional Insight: Omega-3 supplements, such as fish oil or algal oil capsules, can help with joint health and inflammation.

Personal Experience: Taking omega-3 pills has aided my recuperation by reducing inflammation after strenuous calisthenics workouts.

Long-Term Sustainability and Individualization

1. Individualized Approach:

Individuals have different nutritional requirements. Nutrition programs must consider aspects such as age, gender, exercise level, and particular calisthenics objectives.

Personal Experience: Through trial and error, I've found a dietary plan that works for my calisthenics objectives, energy requirements, and general health.

2. Stability and adaptability:

Professional Insight: Nutritional consistency is essential, but flexibility is also essential. Long-term sustainability is ensured by adapting nutritional choices depending on changing exercise intensities and goals.

Personal Experience: I've learned to accept dietary flexibility, allowing for occasional pleasures without jeopardizing my overall nutritional goals.

In conclusion, specific dietary measures are critical for maximizing calisthenics performance. A well-rounded approach to nutrition offers the basis for sustained strength, endurance, and recovery, from macronutrient distribution to micronutrient-rich selections, timing considerations, and possible supplementation.

I can speak to the transforming influence of integrating dietary practices with the demands of calisthenics training based on both professional and personal experiences. Adhering to these rules with attention and a tailored touch will not only improve your physical capabilities, but also contribute to a lifelong path of holistic health and well-being.

CHAPTER 7

30-days Calisthenics Workout Plan for Beginners

Week 1

Day 1:

- Warm-up: 5-10 minutes of simple cardio (jumping jacks, in-place running, etc.)
- Bicep curls using a resistance band (3 sets of 10 reps)
- Tricep extensions using resistance bands (3 sets of 10 reps)
- Rows using resistance bands (3 sets of 10 reps)
- Push-ups (3 sets of 10 reps)

If you can't do a push up, try this instead:

- Wall push ups
- Incline push up
- Negative push up
- Plank hold
- Plank shoulder taps

- Mountain climbers

- Walking plankBodyweight squats (3 sets of 10 reps)
- Hold a plank position for 30 seconds.

If you're having trouble with good squat form. Instead, try this.

- Foot movements
- Toe raises
- Rotations of the ankles
- calf raising

Day 2:

- Warm-up: 5-10 minutes of simple cardio (jumping jacks, in-place running, etc.)
- 3 sets of 5 reps of pull ups
- Shoulder press with resistance band (3 sets of 10 reps)
- Leg curls using a resistance band (3 sets of 10 reps)
- Dips (3 sets of 10 reps)
- Lunges (3 sets of 10 reps)
- Hold a side plank for 30 seconds on each side.

Day 3:

- Warm-up: 5-10 minutes of light exercise (jumping jacks, in-place running, etc.)
- Chest flys using a resistance band (3 sets of 10 reps)
- 3 sets of 10 repetitions of resistance band lateral raises
- Pull-aparts using resistance bands (3 sets of 10 repetitions)
- Push ups in the shape of a diamond (3 sets of 10 reps)
- Squat jumps (3 sets of 10 reps)
- Superman hold (30 second hold)

Week 2:

Day 1

- Warm-up: 5-10 minutes of light exercise (jumping jacks, in-place running, etc.)
- Hammer curls using a resistance band (3 sets of 10 reps)
- Overhead tricep extensions with a resistance band (3 sets of 10 repetitions)
- Pull-downs using a resistance band (3 sets of 10 repetitions)

- Push ups on the decline (3 sets of 10 repetitions)
- Squats in the Bulgarian style (3 sets of 10 repetitions per leg)
- Leg raises with a plank (hold for 30 seconds)

Day 2:

- Warm-up: 5-10 minutes of light exercise (jumping jacks, in-place running, etc.)
- 3 sets of 6 repetitions of pull ups
- Front lifts with a resistance band (3 sets of 10 reps)
- Leg press using a resistance band (3 sets of 10 reps)
- Push ups with a narrow grip (3 sets of 10 reps)
- Lunge jumps (3 sets of 10 repetitions per leg)
- Side plank with leg raises (30 second hold on each side)

Day 3:

- Warm-up: 5-10 minutes of light cardio (jumping jacks, in-place running, etc.)
- 3 sets of 10 repetitions of resistance band chest press
- 3 sets of 10 repetitions of resistance band reverse flys
- Curls using a resistance band (3 sets of 10 reps)
- Push ups with a wide grip (3 sets of 10 reps)
- (Hold for 30 seconds) Wall sit

- Bridge hold (30 second hold)

Week 3:

Day 1

- Warm-up: 5-10 minutes of easy exercise (jumping jacks, in-place running, etc.)
- Curls using a resistance band (3 sets of 10 reps)
- Kickbacks with a resistance band (3 sets of 10 reps)
- Pull-ups (3 sets of 7 reps)
- 3 sets of 10 repetitions of pike push ups
- Weighted Bulgarian split squats (3 sets of 10 repetitions per leg)
- Plank with arm and leg lifts (30 seconds)

Day 2:

- Warm-up: 5-10 minutes of easy exercise (jumping jacks, in-place running, etc.)
- Pull-ups using a resistance band (3 sets of 10 reps)
- 3 sets of 10 repetitions of resistance band lateral raises
- Leg curls with a resistance band and a double band (3 sets of 10 reps)
- Push ups with a tight grip (3 sets of 10 reps)

- 3 sets of 10 repetitions per leg of plyometric lunges
- Side plank with hip dip (30 second hold on each side)

Day 3:

- Warm-up: 5-10 minutes of easy exercise (jumping jacks, in-place running, etc.)
- 3 sets of 10 reps of resistance band chest flys with a pause at the top
- 3 sets of 10 repetitions of resistance band rear delt flys with a pause at the top
- Pull-aparts with a pause at the top (3 sets of 10 repetitions)
- 3 sets of 10 repetitions of clap push ups
- Hold for 30 seconds in a wall sit with calf lift.
- Hold a reverse plank position for 30 seconds.

Week 4:

Day 1

- Warm-up: 5-10 minutes of easy exercise (jumping jacks, in-place running, etc.)
- 3 sets of 10 reps of resistance band bicep curls with a pause at the top

- 3 sets of 10 reps of resistance band tricep extensions with a pause at the bottom
- Pull-ups (3 sets of 8 reps)
- Push ups with an arch (3 sets of 10 reps per side)
- Weighted Bulgarian split squats (3 sets of 10 repetitions per leg)
- Plank with a hip twist (30 seconds)

Day 2:

- Warm-up: 5-10 minutes of easy exercise (jumping jacks, in-place running, etc.)
- Slow eccentric pull-ups (3 sets of 5 reps)
- Front rises with a pause at the top of the resistance band (3 sets of 10 reps)
- Leg press with a pause at the bottom (3 sets of 10 reps)
- 3 sets of 10 reps of push ups with feet raised
- Bridge with one leg (3 sets of 10 reps per leg)
- Side plank with leg raise and hip dip (30 seconds per side)

Day 3:

- Warm-up: 5-10 minutes of easy exercise (jumping jacks, in-place running, etc.)

- 3 sets of 10 repetitions of resistance band chest press with pause at bottom
- 3 sets of 10 reps of resistance band reverse flys with a pause at the top
- Slow eccentric resistance band curls (3 sets of 10 reps)
- Push ups in the shape of Spiderman (3 sets of 10 repetitions per side)
- Knee pulse on the wall (hold for 30 seconds)
- Knee-to-elbow plank (hold for 30 seconds)

Week 5:

Day 1

- Warm-up: 5-10 minutes of easy exercise (jumping jacks, in-place running, etc.)
- 3 sets of 5 reps of pull-ups with an isometric hold at the top
- Slow eccentric lateral lifts with a resistance band (3 sets of 10 reps)
- Squats with a pause at the bottom (3 sets of 10 reps)
- Push ups in the shape of a diamond (3 sets of 10 reps)

- Squats with a leap and pulse at the bottom (3 sets of 10 reps per leg)
- Hold a plank with a hip drop for 30 seconds on each side.

Day 2:

- Warm-up: 5-10 minutes of easy exercise (jumping jacks, in-place running, etc.)
- Slow eccentric resistance band pull-ups (3 sets of 5 reps)
- Leg curls with a resistance band and an isometric hold (3 sets of 10 reps)
- Push-ups with a pause at the bottom (3 sets of 10 reps)
- Jump plyometric lunges (3 sets of 10 repetitions per leg)
- Deadlift with one leg (3 sets of 10 repetitions per leg)
- Side plank with leg raise and knee pulse (30 seconds per side)

Day 3:

- Warm-up: 5-10 minutes of easy exercise (jumping jacks, in-place running, etc.)

- 3 sets of 10 reps of resistance band chest flys with an isometric hold at the top
- Slow eccentric resistance band pull-aparts (3 sets of 10 reps)
- Hammer curls using a resistance band (3 sets of 10 reps)
- Push-ups plyometrically (3 sets of 10 reps)
- Hold for 30 seconds in a wall sit with a heel raise.
- Reach plank (hold for 30 seconds on each side)

CHAPTER 8

7-Day Beginner Calisthenics Meal Plan

Day 1

Breakfast: Scrambled Eggs with Spinach

Ingredients:

- 2 eggs
- a bunch of fresh spinach
- Season with salt and pepper to taste.

Instructions:

1. In a mixing dish, whisk together the eggs.
2. Preheat a nonstick skillet over medium heat.
3. Cook for a minute after adding the spinach.
4. Pour the eggs on top of the spinach.
5. Cook the eggs until they are set.
6. Season with salt and pepper to taste.

Lunch: Salad with grilled chicken

Ingredients:

- Grilled chicken breast
- Greens, mixed
- Tomatoes in the shape of cherries
- Dressing: balsamic vinaigrette

Instructions:

- Cut the grilled chicken breast into slices.
- Toss with mixed greens and cherry tomatoes before serving.
- Dress with the balsamic vinaigrette.

Dinner: Baked Salmon with Quinoa

Ingredients:

- Salmon fillet.
- Quinoa
- Lemon juice steamed broccoli
- Extra virgin olive oil
- seasoned with salt & pepper

Instructions:

- Season the salmon with lemon juice, olive oil, salt, and pepper to taste.
- Once the salmon flakes easily, bake it.
- Serve with steamed broccoli and cooked quinoa.

Snack: Greek Yogurt with Berries

Ingredients:

- Greek yogurt
- Fresh berries, such as raspberries, strawberries, and blueberries

Instructions:

- Put a serving of Greek yogurt in a dish and set it aside.
- The fresh berries should be washed and prepared.
- Serve the Greek yogurt with fresh berries on top.
- Combine them or savor them in layers.
- It's a simple, protein-rich snack with a fruity blast!

Day 2

Breakfast: Oatmeal with Almonds and Honey

Ingredients:

- Rolled oats,
- Almonds, and
- Honey

Instructions:

- Cook the rolled oats according per package directions.
- Drizzle with honey and top with sliced almonds.

Lunch: Turkey and Avocado Wrap

Ingredients:

- whole-grain tortilla
- turkey slices avocado slices
- Greens with a lot of leaves
- (Optional) mustard or mild mayonnaise

Instructions:

1. Spread the tortilla out.

2. Place the turkey, avocado, and leafy leaves on top.
3. If desired, season with mustard or mild mayonnaise.
4. Roll it up and eat it!

Dinner: Stir-Fry of Chickpeas and Vegetables

Ingredients:

- Chickpeas.
- Mixed veggies, such as carrots, broccoli, and bell peppers
- Teriyaki sauce or soy sauce
- Brown rice, cooked

Instructions:

1. Stir-fry the mixed veggies in a wok or pan until they are soft.
2. Add chickpeas and a splash of soy or teriyaki sauce to taste.
3. Over cooked brown rice, serve.

Snack: Sliced Cucumbers with Hummus

Ingredients:

- fresh cucumbers

- Hummus (purchased or homemade)
- Optional (lemon juice)
- Optional seasonings: salt & pepper

Instructions:

1. Clean and thinly slice fresh cucumbers into sticks or rounds.
2. Place the cucumber slices on a serving platter.
3. Serve with hummus on the side for dipping.
4. Squeeze a dab of fresh lemon juice over the cucumbers and season with salt and pepper to taste.
5. This snack combines a crisp crunch with a creamy dip.

Day 3

Breakfast: Whole-Grain Pancakes with Blueberries

Ingredients:

- Whole-Grain Pancakes with Blueberries
- Pancake mix made with whole grains
- Blueberries, fresh
- Optional (optional) maple syrup

Instructions:

1. Cook the pancakes according to package directions.
2. If preferred, top with fresh blueberries and a dab of maple syrup.

Lunch: Tuna Salad

Ingredients:

- Canned tuna
- Greens, mixed Tomatoes in the shape of cherries
- Dressing with olive oil and balsamic vinegar

Instructions:

1. Drain the tuna from the can.
2. Toss with mixed greens and cherry tomatoes before serving.
3. Dress with olive oil and balsamic vinaigrette.

Dinner: Grilled Shrimp with Brown Rice

Ingredients:

- Shrimp
- Brown rice, cooked

- spinach sautéed

Instructions:

1. The shrimp should be grilled until they become pink and start to caramelize.
2. Serve with sautéed spinach on the side and over a bed of cooked brown rice.

Snack: Sliced Apples with Peanut Butter

Ingredients:

- Fresh apples
- Peanut butter (or, if you like, almond butter)

Instructions:

1. Wash and thinly slice fresh apples to make narrow wedges.
2. Serve with peanut butter on the side for dipping.
3. Simply dip an apple slice into the peanut butter and enjoy the sweet and nutty tastes.
4. It's a traditional and filling snack.

Day 4

Breakfast: Greek Yogurt with Granola and Banana

Ingredients:

- Greek yogurt
- Granola
- slices of banana

Instructions:

- In a mixing dish, layer Greek yogurt, granola, and sliced banana.

Lunch: Salad with Quinoa and Black Beans

Ingredients:

- Cooked quinoa
- Beans, black
- Bell peppers, chopped
- Dressing: lime vinaigrette

Instructions:

1. Combine the quinoa, black beans, and sliced bell peppers.

2. Toss with the lime vinaigrette dressing.

Dinner: Baked Chicken Thighs with Sweet Potatoes

Ingredients:

- Chicken thighs
- Yummy sweet potatoes
- Garlic, rosemary, and olive oil

Instructions:

- Olive oil, garlic, and rosemary season chicken thighs.
- Bake until the chicken is done and the sweet potatoes are soft.

Snack: Carrot Sticks with Hummus

Ingredients:

- Fresh carrots Hummus (either store-bought or homemade)
- Optional seasonings: salt & pepper

Instructions:

1. Fresh carrots should be washed and peeled.
2. Carrots can be cut into sticks or slices.
3. Serve the carrot sticks with hummus on the side.
4. For added taste, season with a touch of salt and pepper.
5. Enjoy this crispy and healthy snack!

Day 5

Breakfast: Scrambled Tofu with Spinach

Ingredients:

- Tofu, fresh spinach, onion, and garlic
- Turmeric (to add color)
- seasoned with salt & pepper

Instructions:

1. To begin, crumble the tofu into a basin.
2. In a skillet, sauté chopped onion and garlic until transparent.
3. Combine the crumbled tofu, turmeric, salt, and pepper in a mixing bowl. Cook until well heated.
4. Cook until the spinach has wilted.

Lunch: Spinach and Feta Stuffed Chicken Breast

Ingredients:

- Chicken thigh
- Feta cheese and fresh spinach
- Spices, olive oil, and lemon juice

Instructions:

1. The chicken breast should be butterflyed.
2. Stuff with feta cheese and fresh spinach.
3. Drizzle with olive oil, lemon juice, and seasonings of choice.
4. Bake the chicken until it is done.

Dinner: Baked Cod with Asparagus

Ingredients:

- cod fillet
- asparagus
- lemon juice
- garlic and
- herbs.

Instructions

1. Season the fish with lemon juice, garlic, and herbs of your choosing.
2. Arrange the asparagus on a baking pan, then top with the fish.
3. Bake until the cod readily flakes.

Snack: Mixed Nuts

Ingredients:

- Assorted mixed nuts (almonds, walnuts, cashews)

Instructions:

1. Simply grab a handful of your favorite mixed nuts and get to work.
2. There is no further preparation required.
3. Enjoy this nutrient-dense and filling snack with healthy fats and protein.

Day 6

Breakfast: Protein Smoothie

Ingredients:

- Protein powder
- Almond
- banana milk

Instructions:

1. Blend the protein powder, a banana, and almond milk until smooth.

Lunch: Lentil Soup

Ingredients

- Cooked lentils
- Vegetable mixture
- Spices Vegetable broth

Instructions:

2. For a substantial soup, simmer cooked lentils, mixed veggies, vegetable broth, and seasonings.

Dinner: Grilled Portobello Mushrooms with Quinoa

Ingredients:

- Portobello mushrooms
- Olive oil and
- quinoa balsamic vinegar

Instructions:

3. Blend balsamic vinegar and olive oil to marinate portobello mushrooms.
4. Grill until the meat is tender.
5. Serve with quinoa that has been cooked.

Snack: Guacamole-topped sliced peppers

Ingredients:

- Fresh bell peppers (select a variety of hues for visual appeal)
- Guacamole (purchased or prepared from scratch)

Instructions:

1. Wash and thinly slice fresh bell peppers into strips or sticks.
2. On a platter, arrange the pepper strips.
3. Serve with guacamole for dipping on the side.

4. Dip a pepper strip into the guacamole and enjoy the creamy, somewhat spicy flavor combo.
5. This snack has a variety of textures and tastes.

Day 7

Breakfast: Cottage Cheese with Pineapple

Ingredients:

- Cottage cheese
- pineapple slices, fresh

Instructions:

1. Serve the cottage cheese with fresh pineapple pieces.

Lunch: Roast Turkey and Veggie Bowl

Ingredients:

- Slices of roasted turkey
- roasted veggies assortment
- Sauce or light gravy

Instructions:

2. Mix pieces of roast turkey with other roasted veggies.
3. Drizzle lightly with gravy or sauce.

Dinner: Baked Tilapia with Green Beans

Ingredients:

- Tilapia fillet
- green beans
- lemon juice
- garlic and
- herbs

Instructions:

1. Add your preferred herbs, garlic, and lemon juice to the fish.
2. Bake until the fish readily flakes.
3. Serve alongside steaming green beans.

Snack: Mixed Berries

Ingredients:

- A variety of fresh berries, such as blackberries, raspberries, blueberries, and strawberries

Instructions:

1. Gently pat the mixed berries with a paper towel after giving them a good wash and letting them dry.
2. Put the berries in a basin or container.
3. Fresh mixed berries are a simple and delicious snack. There are no additional ingredients or preparation required!

Conclusion

Congratulations on learning about the importance of nutrition in your bodyweight workout adventure. It's not just about sweat and effort; it's about feeding your body to push yourself to new limits.

Keep in mind that nutrition is your hidden weapon. Create a meal plan that is specific to your objectives and interests, balancing protein, carbohydrates, and healthy fats.

It is critical to time your pre- and post-workout meals. Make use of these ways to boost your performance and recuperation.

Your food plan is an ally, not a constraint. Accept it, appreciate it, and incorporate it into your regular routine.

Keep pushing your limitations and savoring each win as you continue your bodyweight training experience. Your success is defined not only by physical improvements, but also by discipline, resilience, and devotion.

You write your own tale, and nutrition is the ink that makes it come to life. So, keep going, stay focused, and make your bodyweight exercises the most fantastic experience of your life. On to the next adventure.